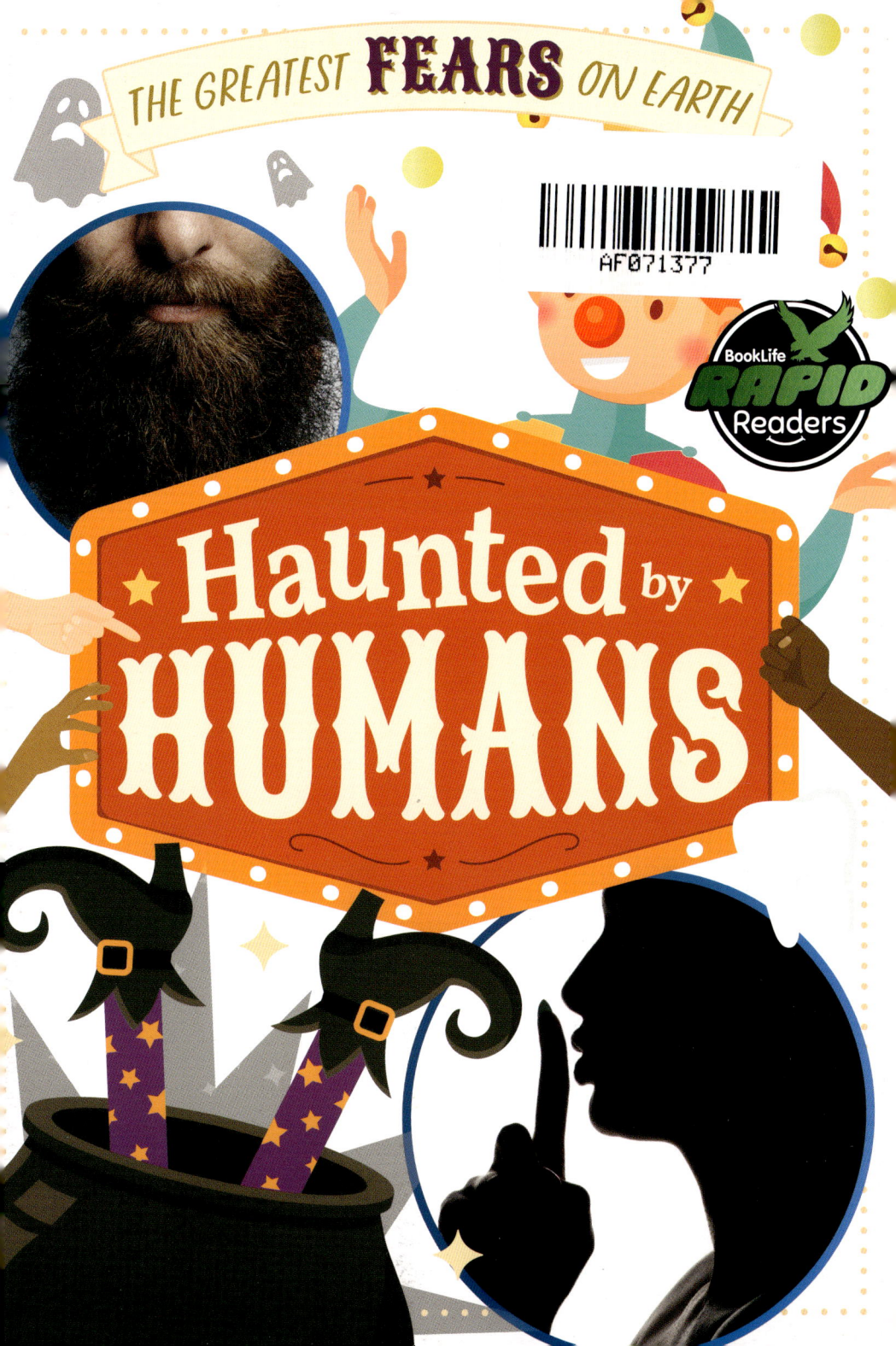

BookLife PUBLISHING

©2023
BookLife Publishing Ltd.
King's Lynn, Norfolk
PE30 4LS, UK

All rights reserved.
Printed in China.

A catalogue record for this book is available from the British Library.

ISBN: 978-1-80505-030-8

Written by:
John Wood
Adapted by:
Noah Leatherland
Edited by:
Kirsty Holmes
Designed by:
Isabella Croker

FSC® C113515 — MIX Paper from responsible sources — www.fsc.org

All facts, statistics, web addresses and URLs in this book were verified as valid and accurate at time of writing. No responsibility for any changes to external websites or references can be accepted by either the author or publisher.

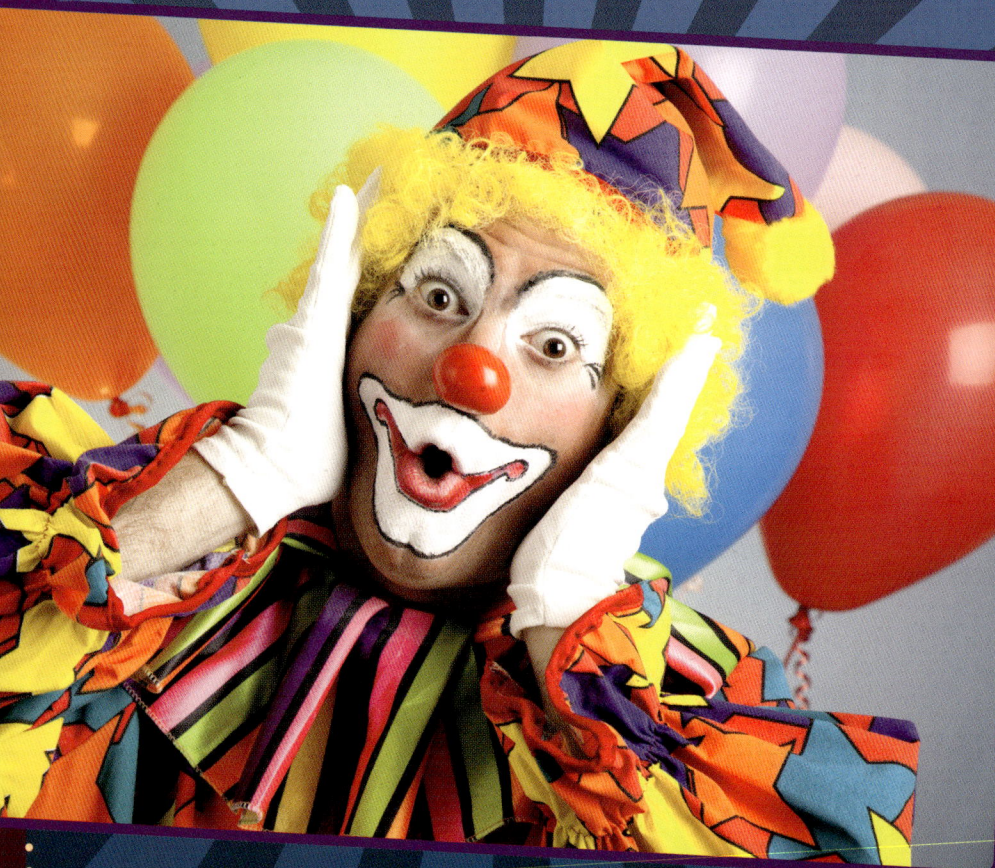

Photo Credits

Images are courtesy of Shutterstock.com. With thanks to Getty Images, Thinkstock Photo and iStockphoto.
RECURRING – Denys Koltovskyi, vectorlight, v_v_v, pikepicture. COVER – Vladimir Gjorgiev, vectorlight, Denys Koltovskyi, ONYXprj, Ground Picture, Tartila, v_v_v. 4–5 – The Faces, sicegame. 6–7 – Evgeniya Litovchenko, VectorPunks, Hohum. 8–9 – Enrique Romero, Sarah Guilford. 10–11 – andriano.cz, Nick Hawkes. 12–13 – sciencepics, Kateryna Kon. 14–15 – icon0.com, lingdamphotothailand, karelnoppe, iconriver, Gavrilo Stanojevic. 16–17 – Alex Mit, klyots, Anastasi17. 18–19 – Shuravaya, viviana loza, GoodStudio. 20–21 – Terdsak L, LightField Studios, C Design Studio. 22–23 – Lemonreader, 995577823Xyn (WikiCommons). 24–25 – Pavel Krasensky, Prostock-studio, WinWin artlab. 26–27 – Lisa F. Young, nito. 28–29 – Torychemistry, UfaBizPhoto, YummyBuum. 30–31 – pikepicture.

CONTENTS

*Words that look like **this** are explained in the glossary on page 31.*

Page 4 Welcome to the Show!
Page 6 Wicked Witches
Page 8 Beastly Beards
Page 10 Nasty Knees
Page 12 The Science of Fear
Page 16 Teeth of Terror
Page 18 Cannot Bare It!
Page 20 Scared Speechless
Page 22 Our Guest Star
Page 24 Evil Itching
Page 26 Creepy Clowns
Page 28 A Phobia of Phobias?
Page 30 Curtain Close
Page 31 Glossary
Page 32 Index

WELCOME TO THE SHOW!

"COME ONE, COME ALL! COME AND SEE SOME OF THE GREATEST FEARS KNOWN TO HUMANITY!"

We have all felt fear in our lives. But do you have a phobia? A phobia is a strong fear of something, such as spiders or flying.

People have phobias of all sorts of things. Some people have phobias of things where there is no real danger.

The things you will see in our show were found all over the world. These are all real fears. Are you ready to find out what scares people the most?

Who knows, maybe you will leave the show with a brand-new phobia of your own?

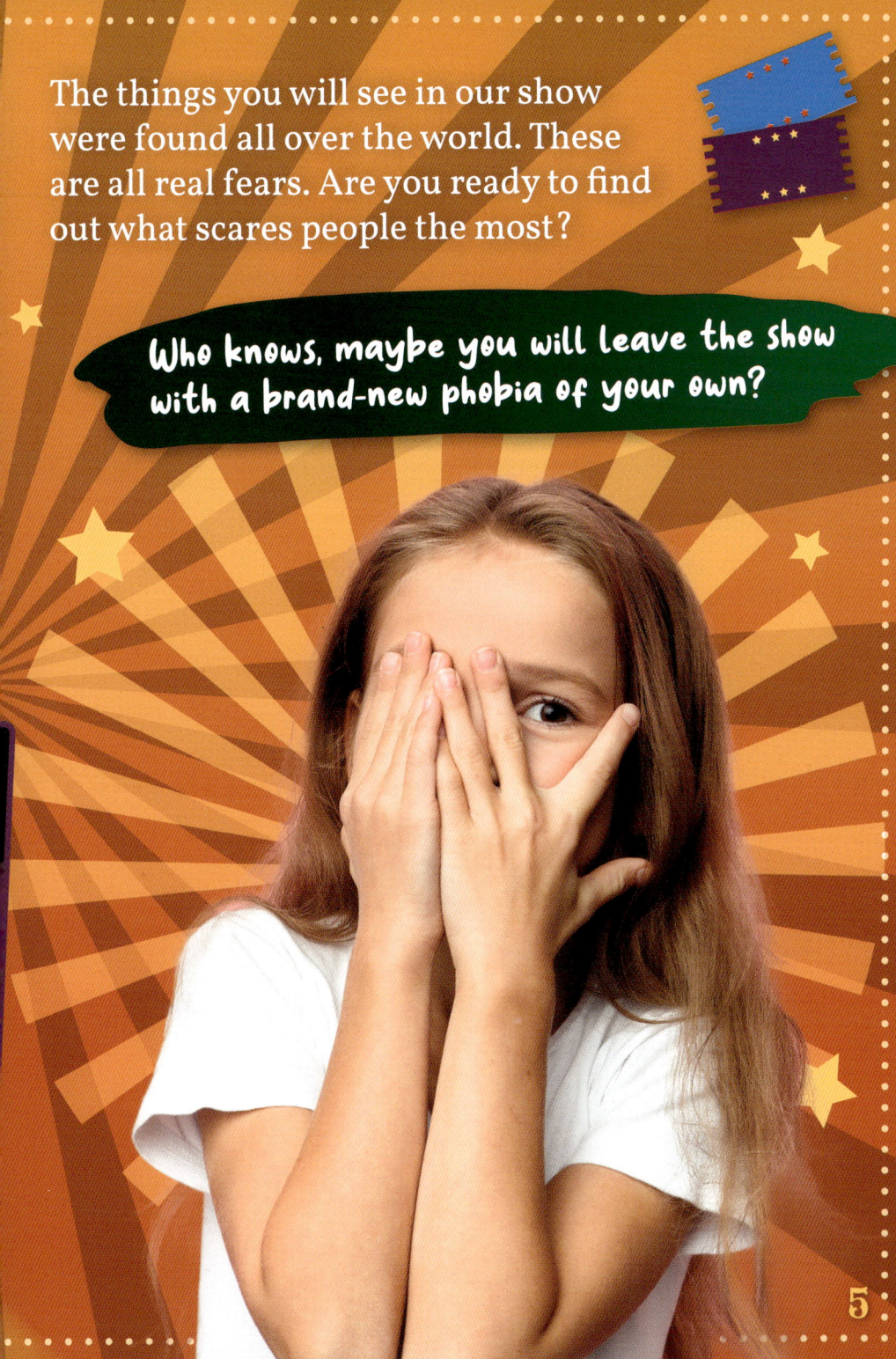

WICKED WITCHES

It comes from the woods... An ugly laugh in the middle of the night. Somewhere in the twisted trees, the witches use their evil magic. They say witches collect all sort of gross **ingredients** for their spells.

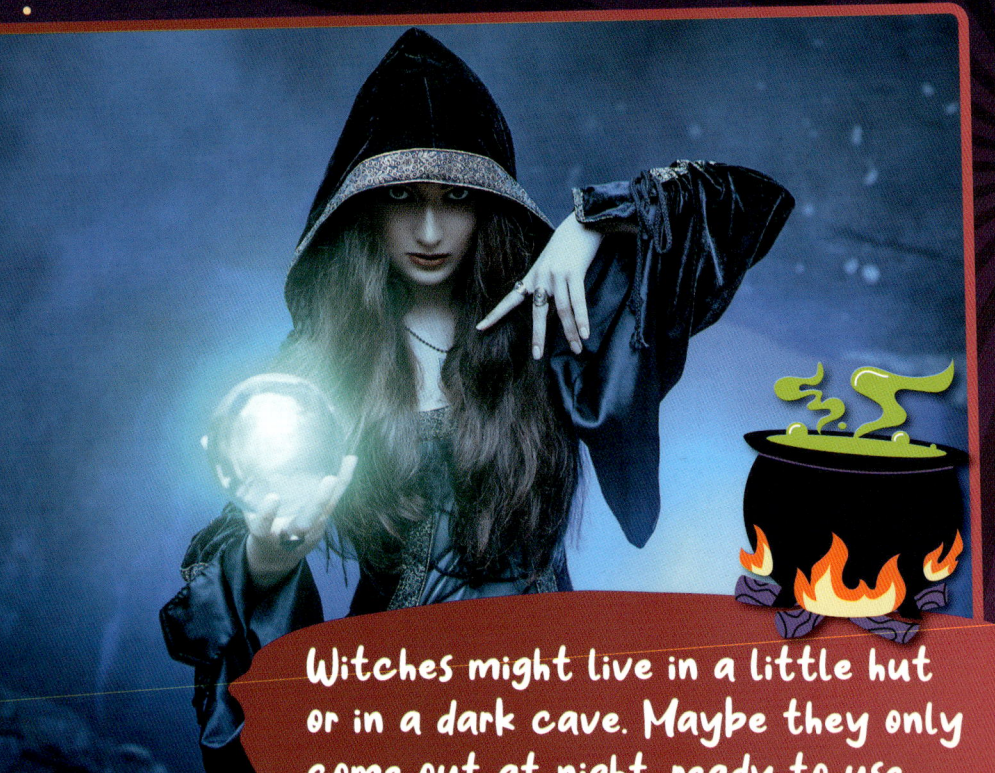

Witches might live in a little hut or in a dark cave. Maybe they only come out at night, ready to use their spells on whoever they find.

Hundreds of years ago, people were very worried. Could people they knew secretly be evil? They were so scared of witches they went on witch hunts.

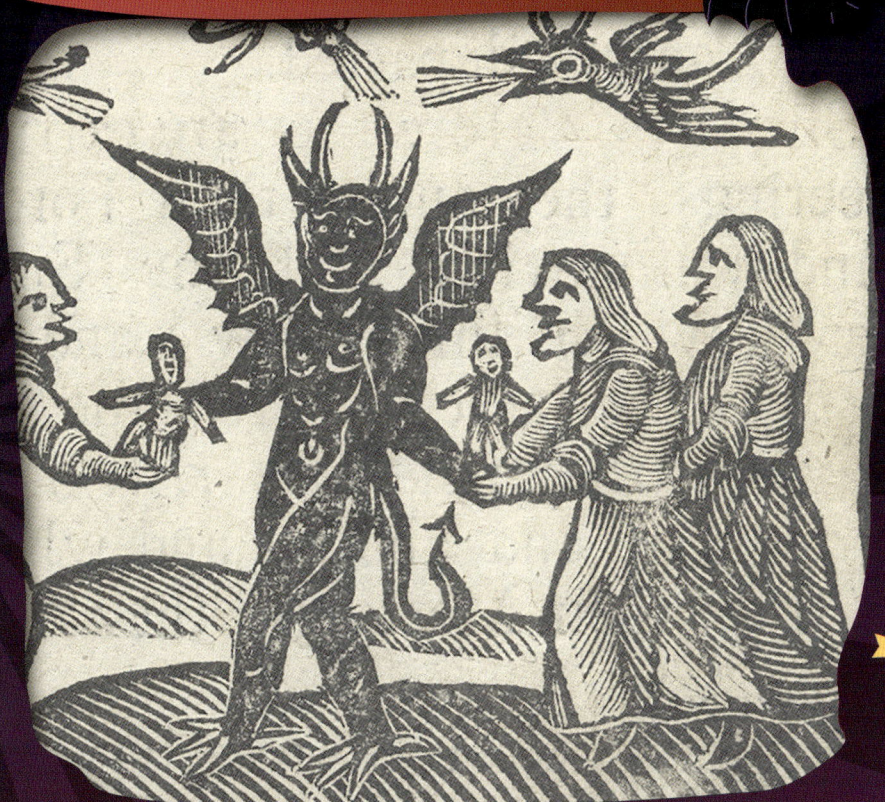

The most famous witch hunt happened in an American town called Salem in 1692 and 1693. It was called the Salem Witch Trials. 150 people were said to be witches. 19 were **executed** and five were put in prison.

BEASTLY BEARDS

Do you know someone with a beard? Someone in your family? Maybe your teacher has one. Is it long and tangled or are the hairs short and rough? Do they scare you?

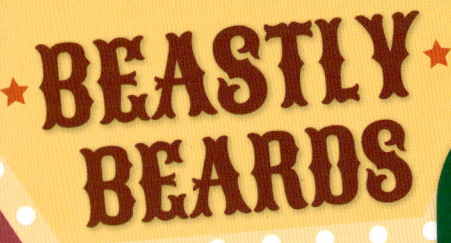

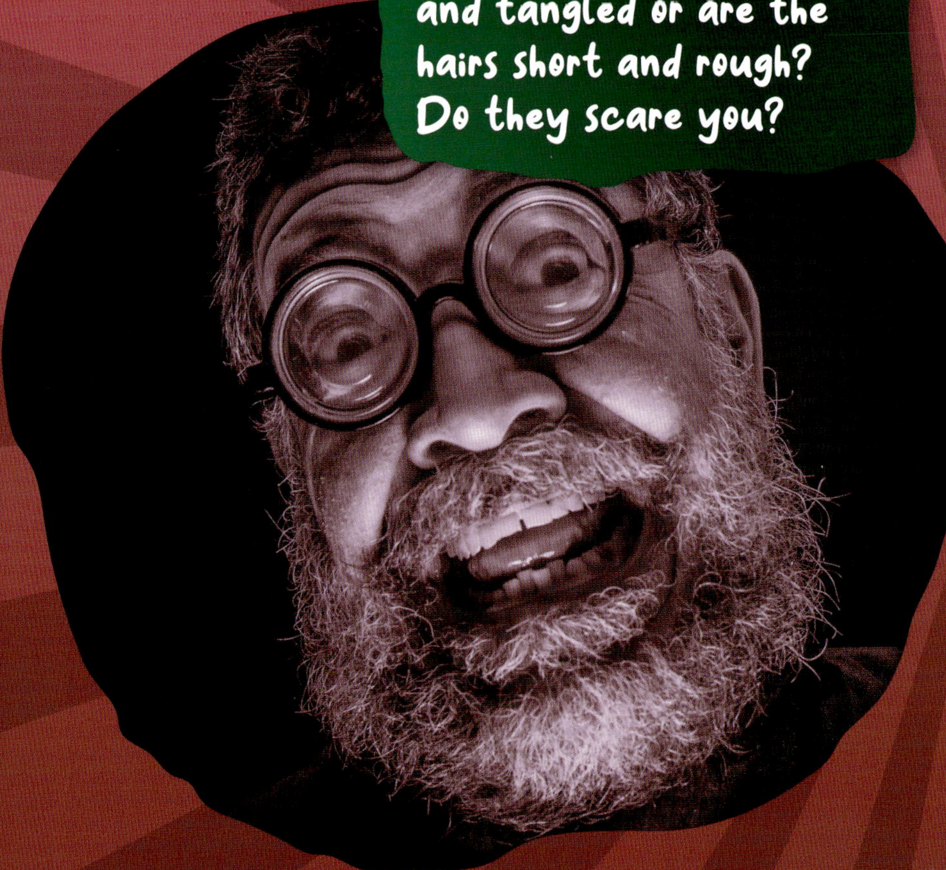

To some people, beards are things to be afraid of. They may seem harmless, but they could have dark secrets.

There are a few reasons why someone might tremble at the sight of a beard. Some people are scared of all the dirt and crumbs that could be mixed in with the hairs.

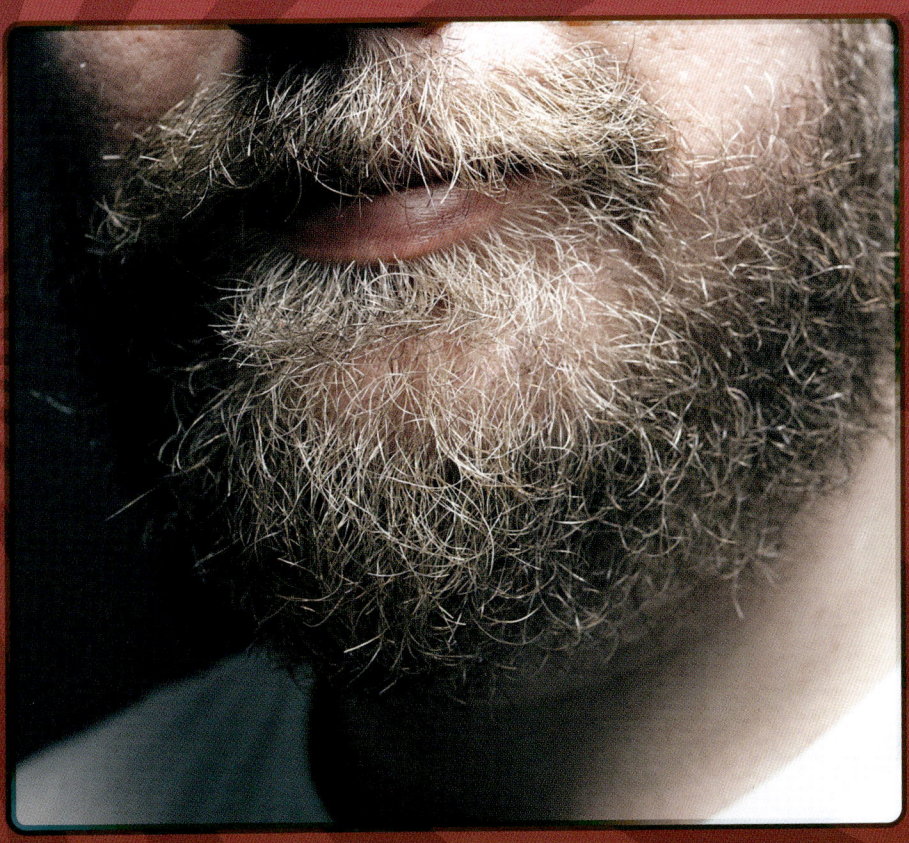

Others are scared of beards because they cover someone's face. What are they hiding? What do they really look like under all that hair?

NASTY KNEES

What do you see when you go to the beach? Anything that scares you? For some people, when the weather gets nice and hot, it is their worst nightmare. That is when the knees come out!

All sorts of knees can scare people. Bony knees, wrinkly knees, big knees, small knees, hairy knees, bruised knees – the horror!

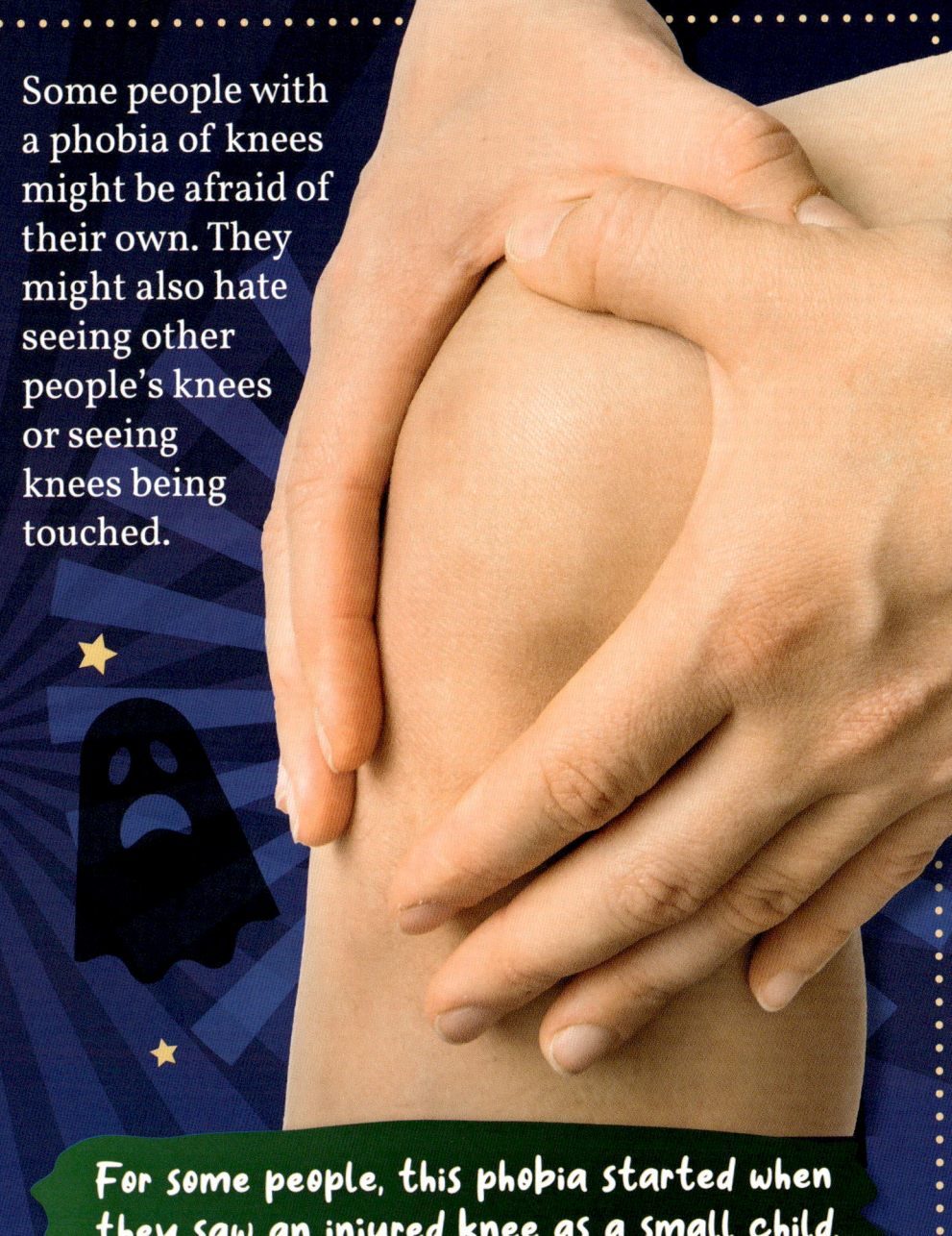

Some people with a phobia of knees might be afraid of their own. They might also hate seeing other people's knees or seeing knees being touched.

For some people, this phobia started when they saw an injured knee as a small child. Look down at you own knees. Touch the wrinkly skin. How do they make you feel?

THE SCIENCE OF FEAR

NERVOUS SYSTEM

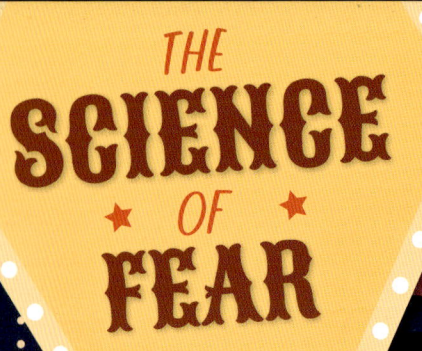

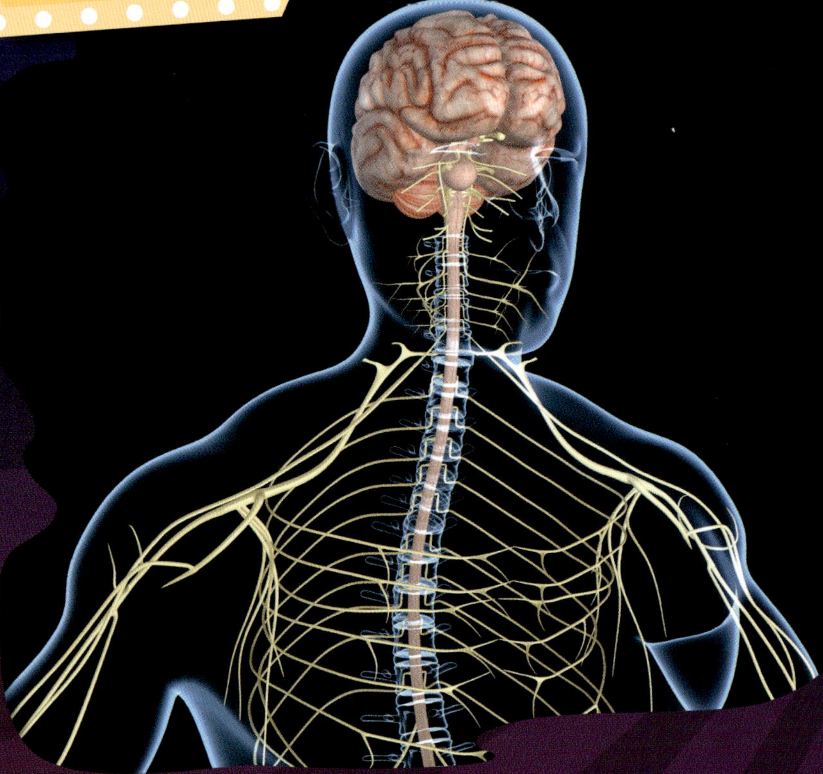

The nervous system is a network of nerves that send messages around your body. Some of these messages are controlled by you, such as moving your arms and legs. Some messages are **automatic**, such as the ones that are sent when you get scared.

Lots of things happen in your body when you are scared. You might sweat and shake. Your breathing and your heart rate will get faster.

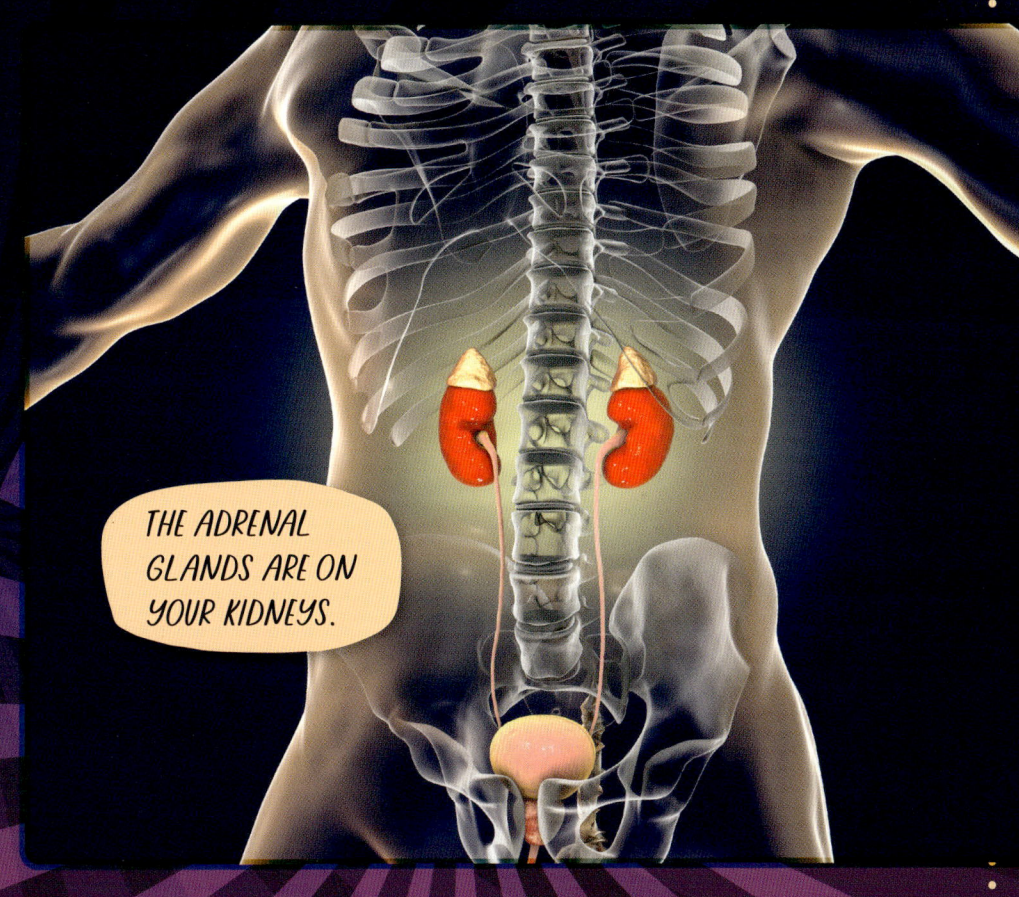

THE ADRENAL GLANDS ARE ON YOUR KIDNEYS.

Your brain also sends a message to your adrenal glands. Glands are parts of the body that release helpful things. The adrenal glands release a <u>hormone</u> called adrenaline.

ADRENALINE

Adrenaline moves through your blood and tells the body to get ready for action. It makes your heart beat faster, your breath quicken and your muscles tense.

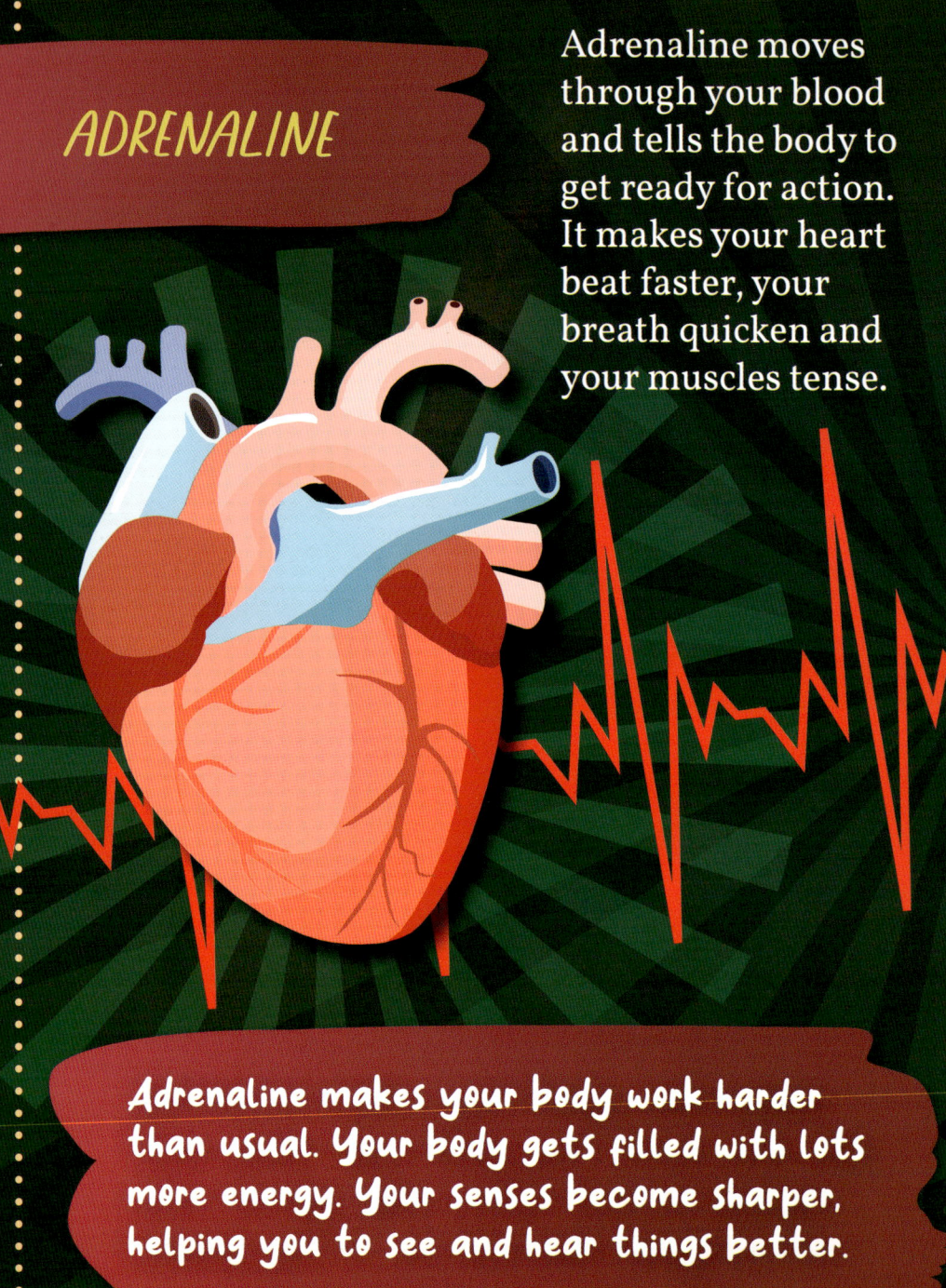

Adrenaline makes your body work harder than usual. Your body gets filled with lots more energy. Your senses become sharper, helping you to see and hear things better.

FALSE ALARM

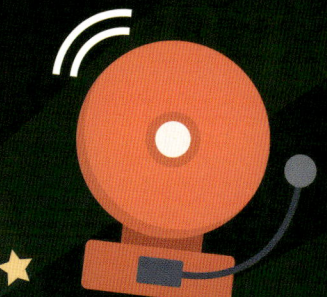

The nervous system is like an alarm for your body. It can alert you when your body is too hot or too cold, hungry or thirsty and when you feel danger.

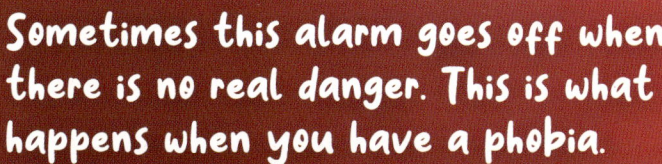

Sometimes this alarm goes off when there is no real danger. This is what happens when you have a phobia.

TEETH OF TERROR

Nobody likes going to the dentist. For some people, it is their worst fear. They hate the feeling of being sat in the dentist's chair, unable to move.

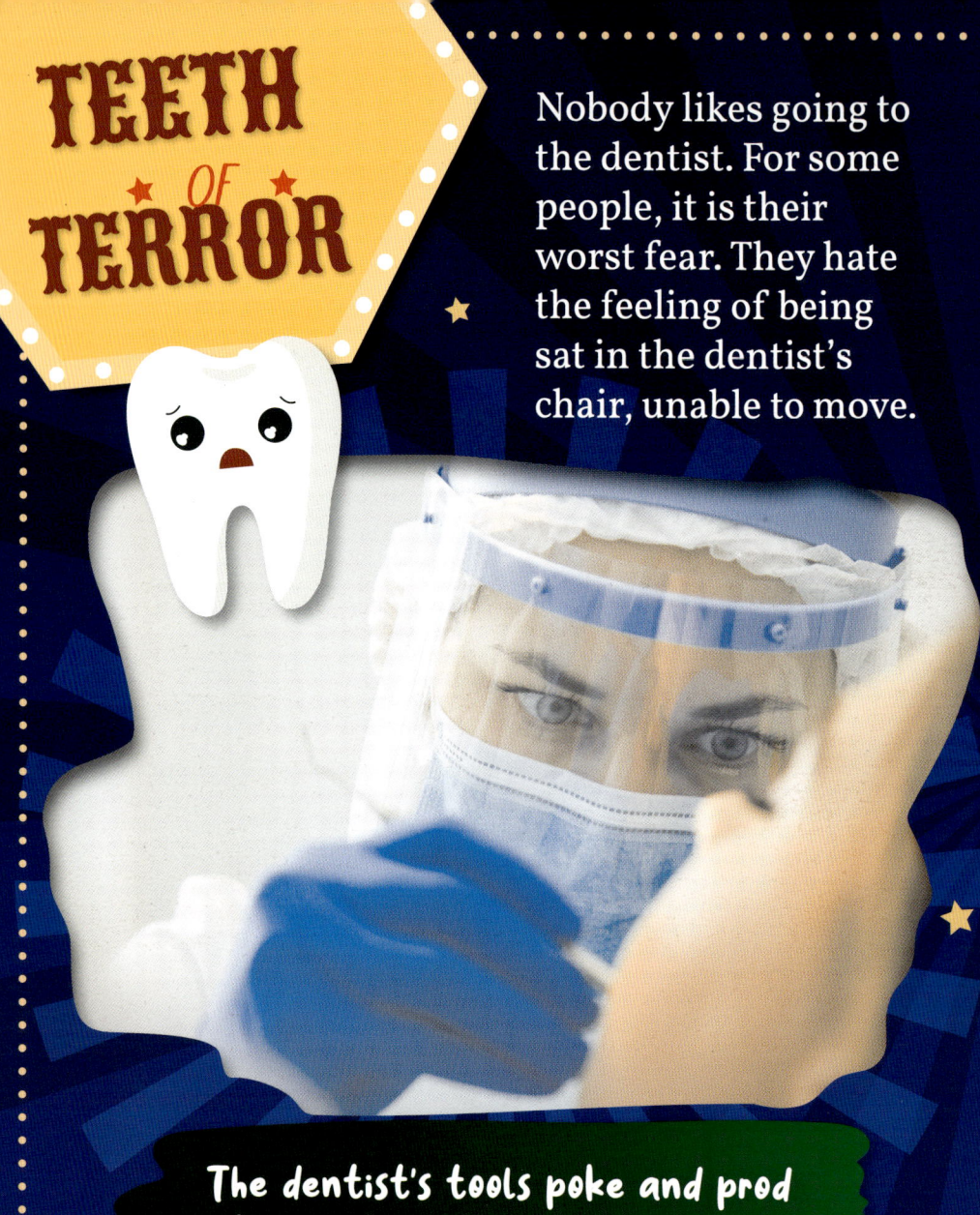

The dentist's tools poke and prod at your teeth and gums. Who knows what they will find in your mouth? What might they take out? What might they put in?

When people have phobia of dentists, they might not get their teeth checked for a long time. This can create big problems with their teeth that can cause a lot of pain.

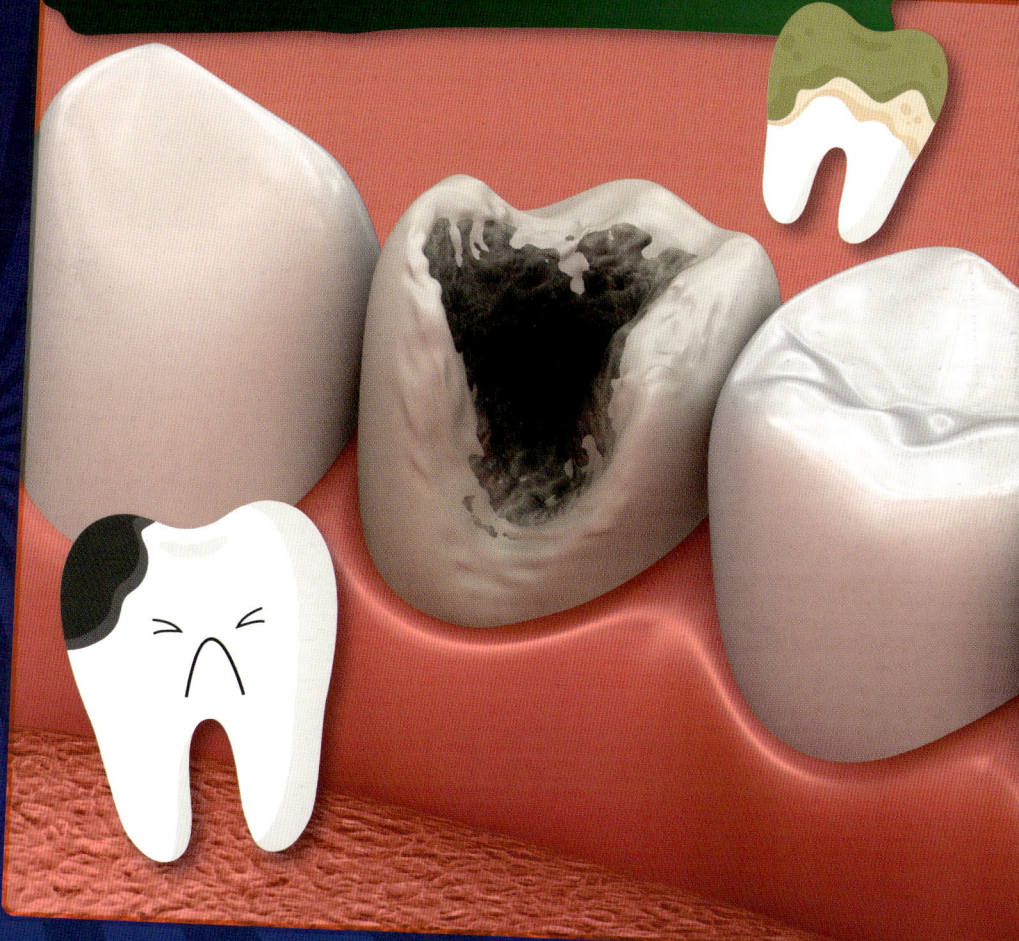

As scary as going to the dentist might be, it is their job to take care of you. They want to help you and your teeth to stay healthy.

CANNOT BARE IT!

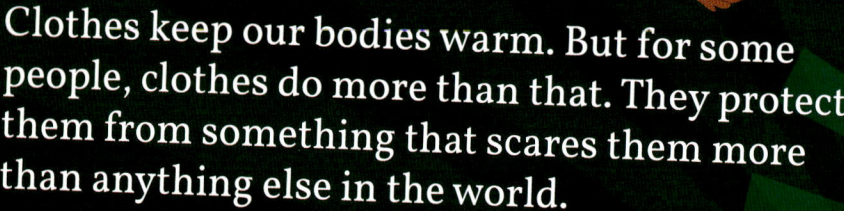

Clothes keep our bodies warm. But for some people, clothes do more than that. They protect them from something that scares them more than anything else in the world.

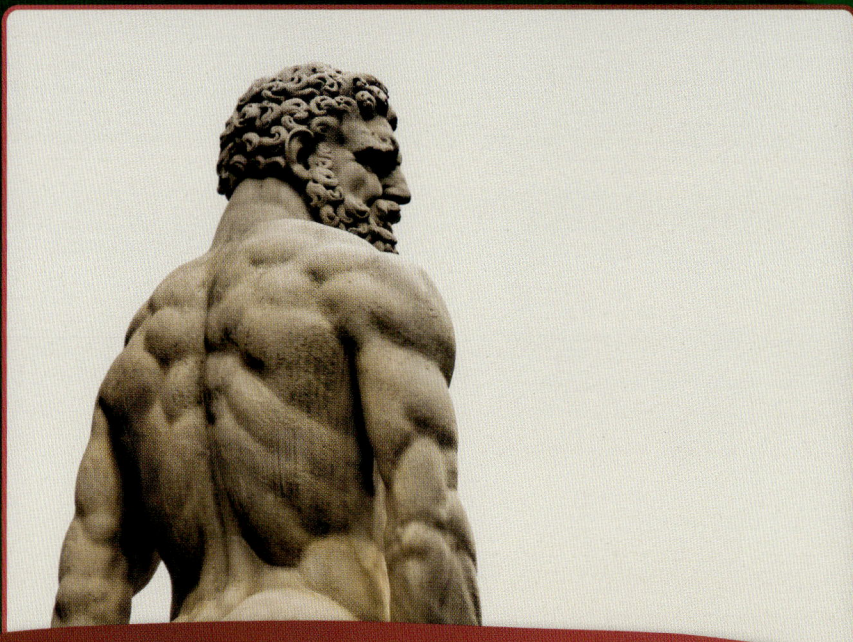

Some people are terrified of being naked. It might be to do with how helpless we might feel when naked. Our bodies are private and being naked leaves us <u>vulnerable</u>.

People with a phobia of nakedness might not like to see themselves naked, or they might be afraid of seeing others naked.

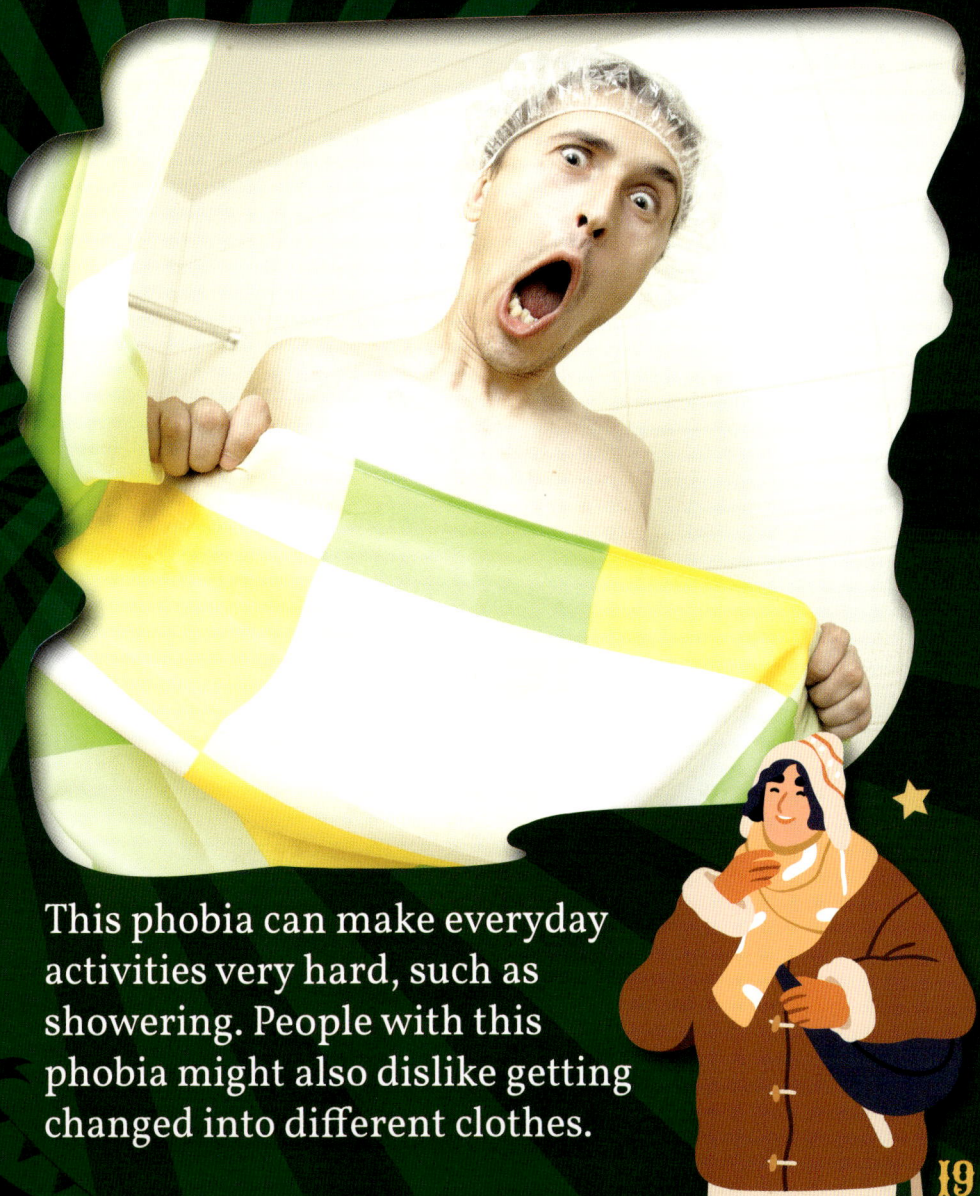

This phobia can make everyday activities very hard, such as showering. People with this phobia might also dislike getting changed into different clothes.

SCARED SPEECHLESS

Do you like to speak in front of crowds? Or does it scare you? All their blank faces and their eyes looking right at you. They are waiting for you to say something. Anything.

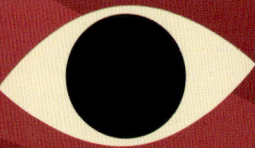

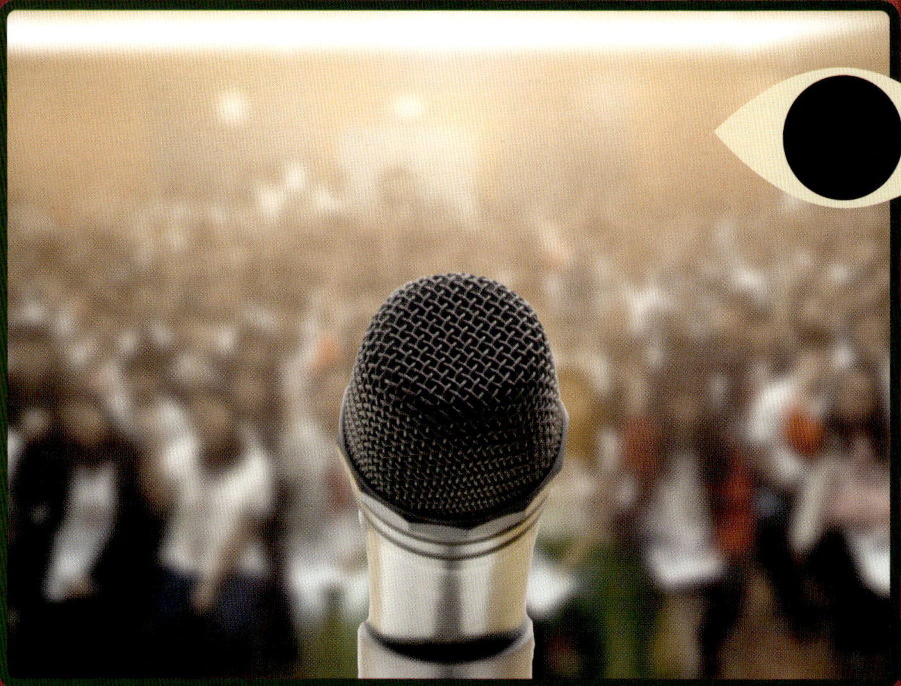

But it is silent. You do not know what to say but they just keep staring at you. It feels like it will never stop.

The fear of speaking in front of people is sometimes called stage fright. It is more common in younger people than older people.

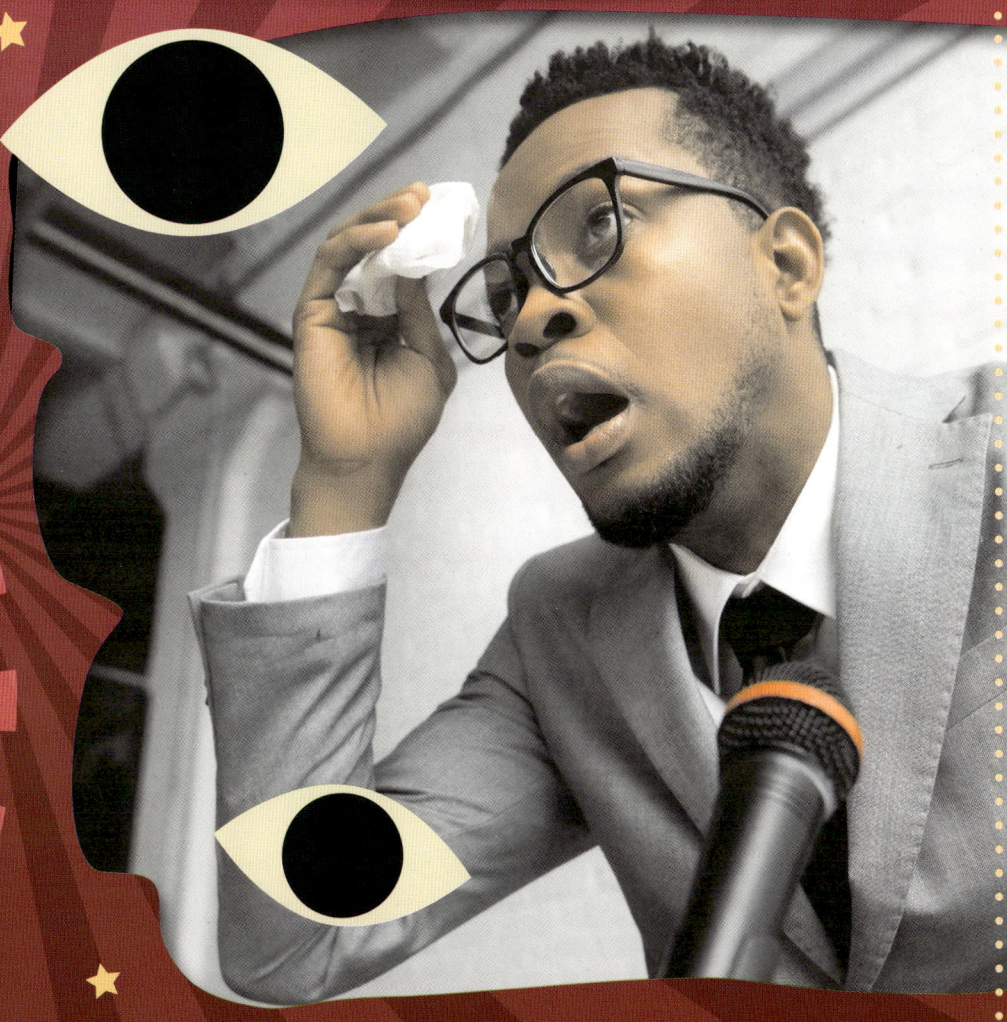

For some people, speaking in front of people is a big part of their jobs. They might get special training to help them with their phobia.

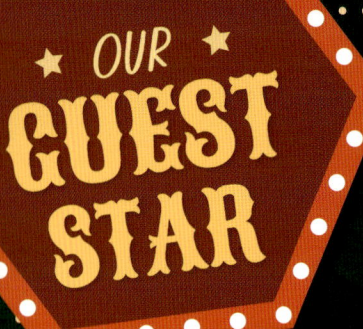

OUR GUEST STAR

Marilyn Monroe was a famous actor and model from the US. She was born in 1926, and had a difficult childhood. Her parents could not look after her, so she was raised in an **orphanage**.

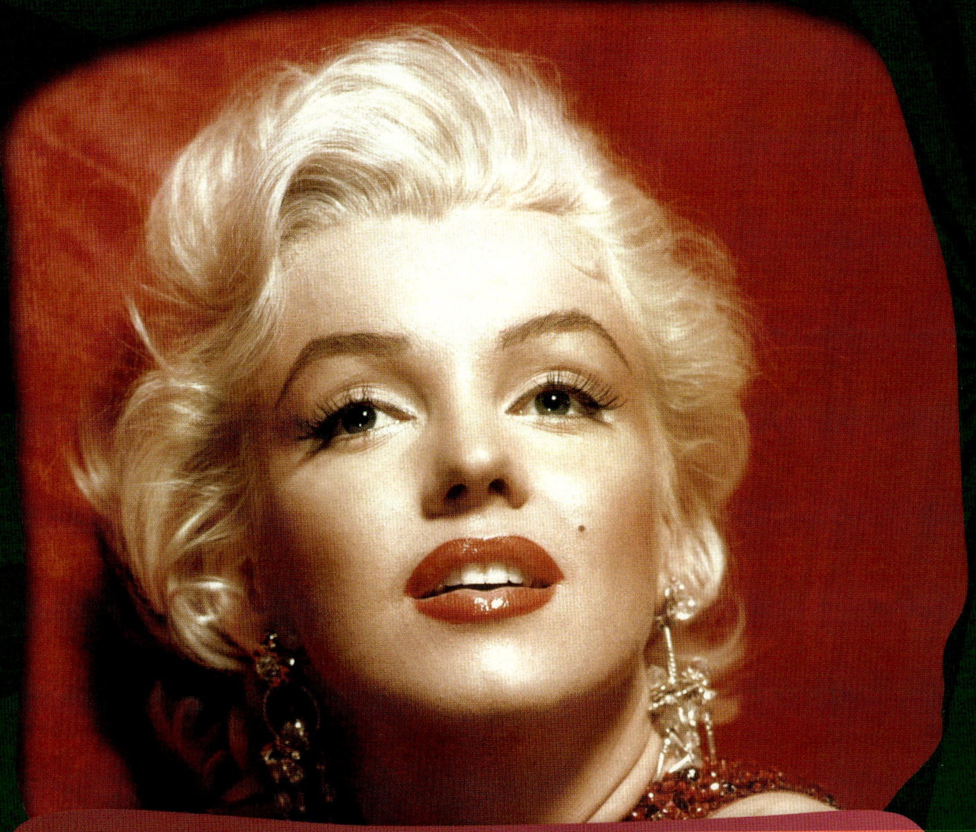

When Marilyn grew up, she starred in 23 films, which earned her millions of dollars. She became one of the most famous people in the US.

Marilyn Monroe had a fear of speaking. Growing up, she spoke with a stutter. This meant that she would say the first sound of a word over and over again and found it hard to say the rest.

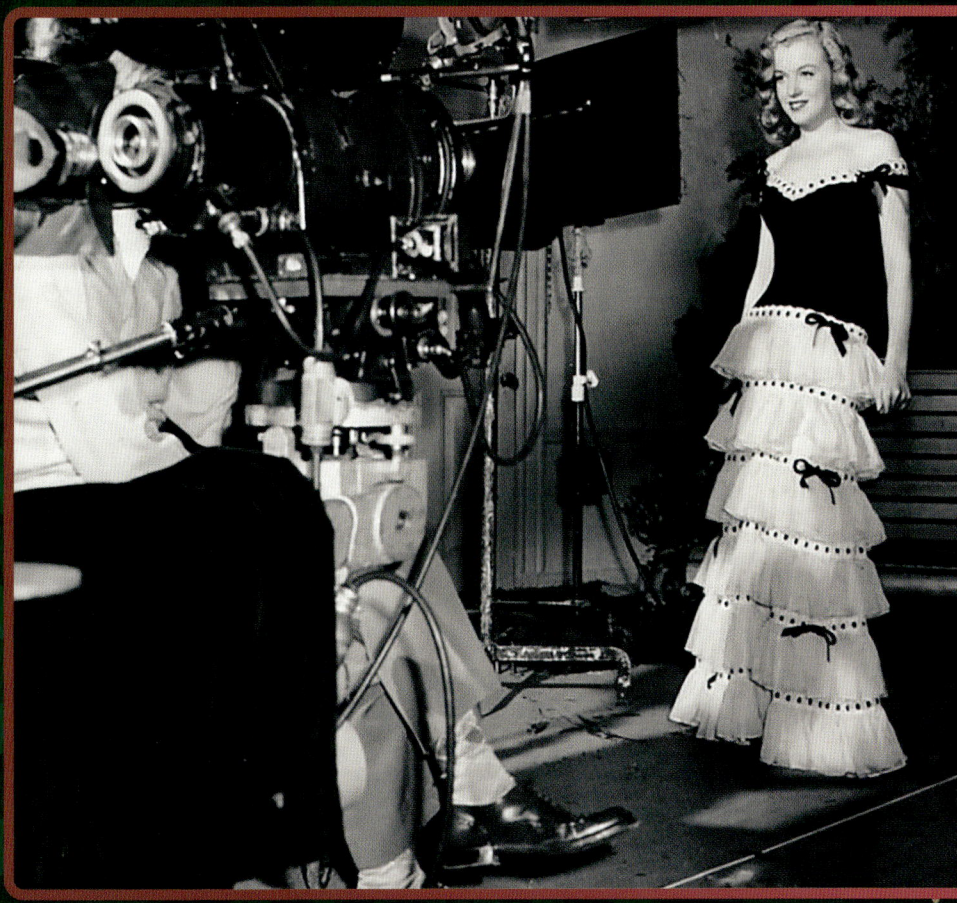

Marilyn managed her phobia by speaking very slowly and carefully. It helped and she became famous for her slow way of talking.

EVIL ITCHING

Do you feel that itch on your arm? Try to ignore it, no matter how much you want to scratch it. Do not do it!

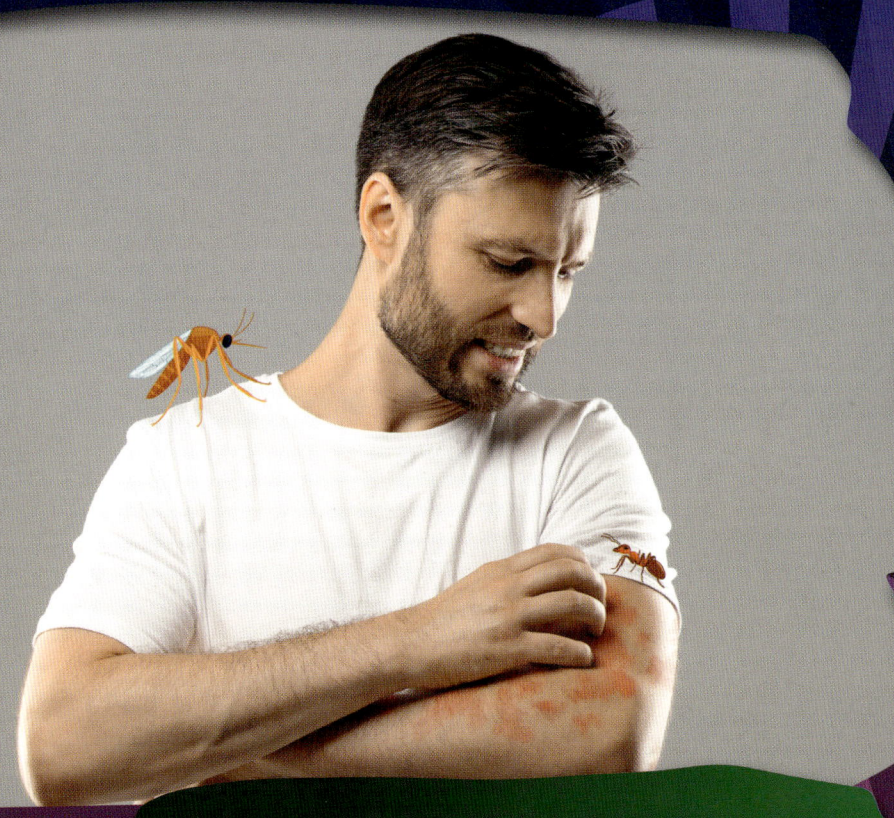

But, what if it is a bug? Maybe it is hundreds of tiny creatures digging into your skin? Now you feel the itch all over your head. Now it is on a spot on your back you cannot reach.

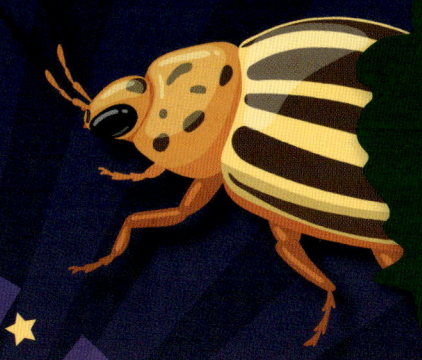

It is very hard not to scratch an itch. This phobia is not just the fear of itching — it is also the fear of bugs that cause itching.

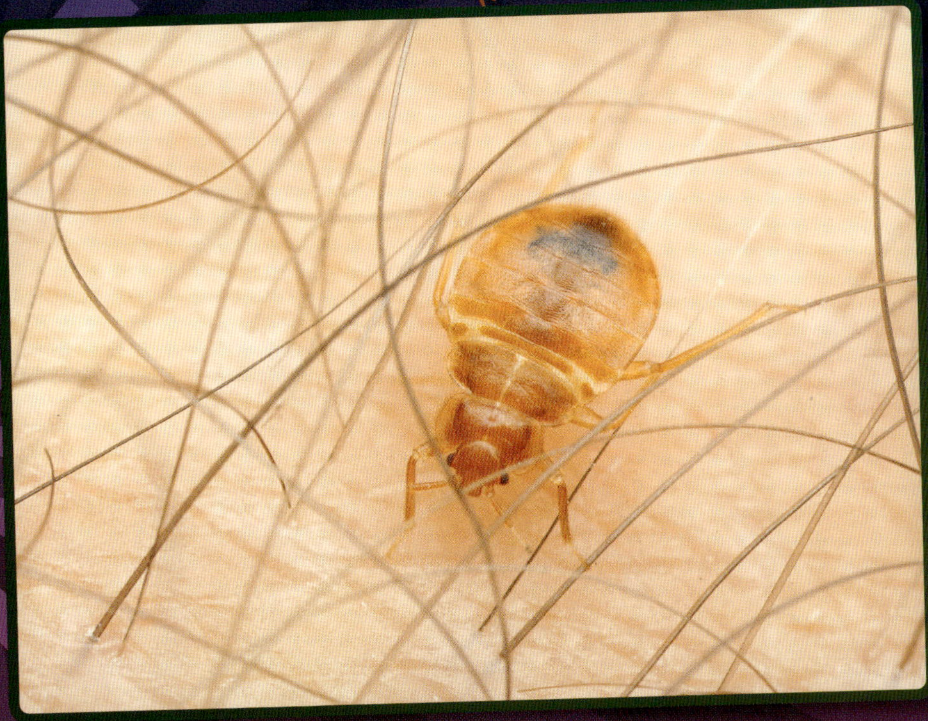

People with this phobia might scratch themselves all the time and constantly clean their homes. Sometimes, just thinking about itching can make you feel a tingle.

CREEPY CLOWNS

Now comes the fun part of our show – bring out the clowns! Their faces are as white as skulls. Their noses are as red as blood. You never know what they are going to do next!

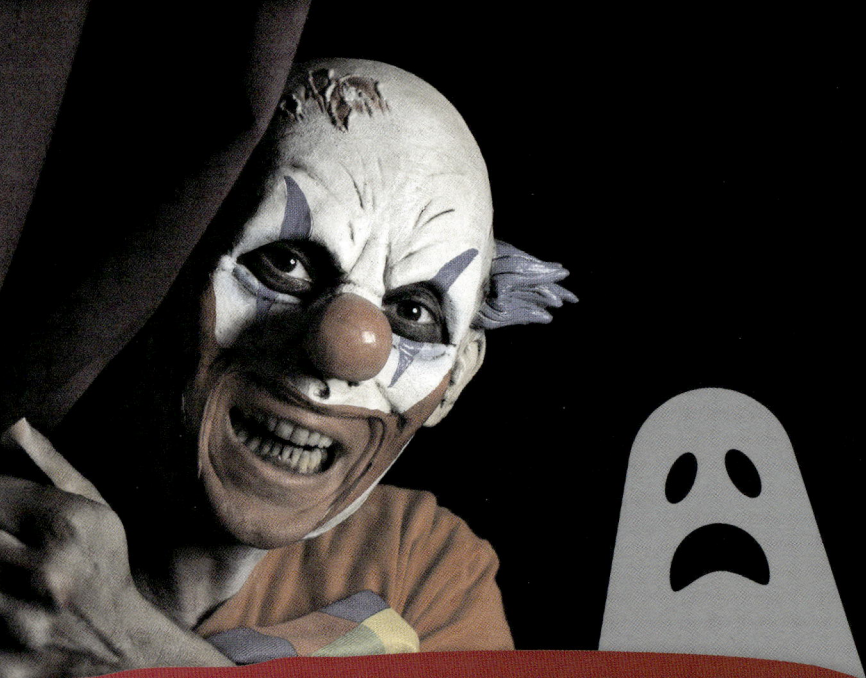

They will make you laugh until you cry... or, maybe they will just make you cry. Who knows what crazy toys they have hidden away?

Clowns have been around for thousands of years. They used to be called jesters, and they would <u>entertain</u> and <u>advise</u> leaders and rulers.

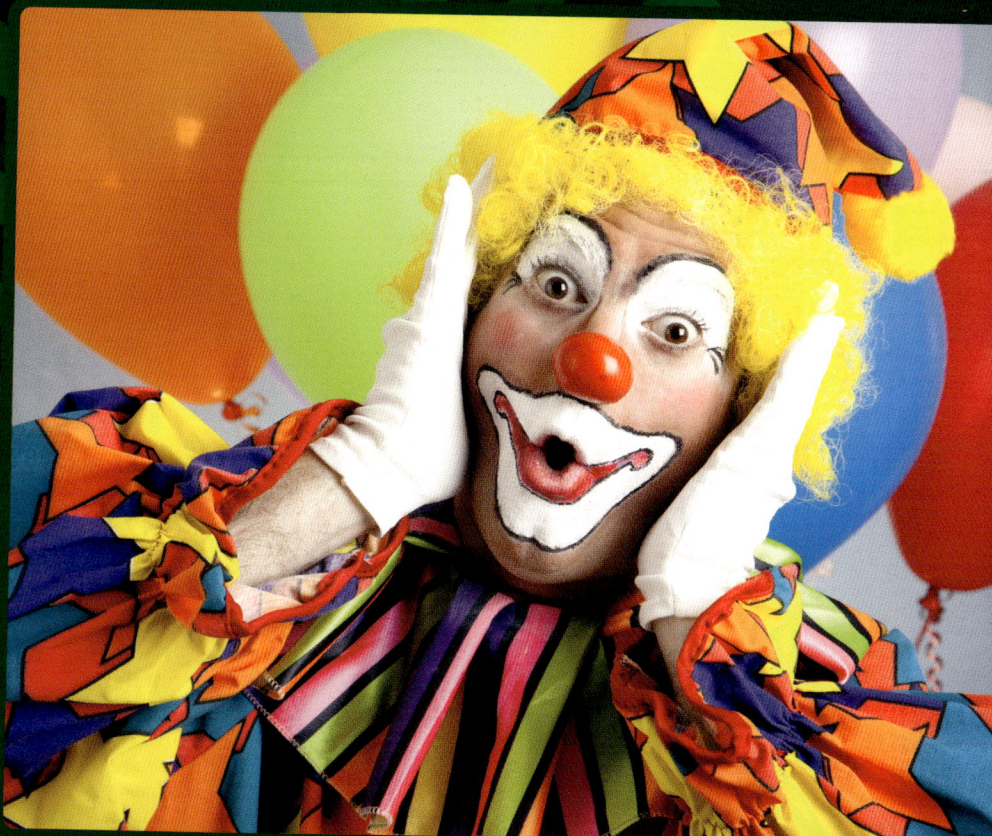

Do you think clowns are creepy? Is it all the make-up that hides their face? Their big curly hair? Why do they hide their real faces? What secrets are they hiding?

A PHOBIA OF PHOBIAS?

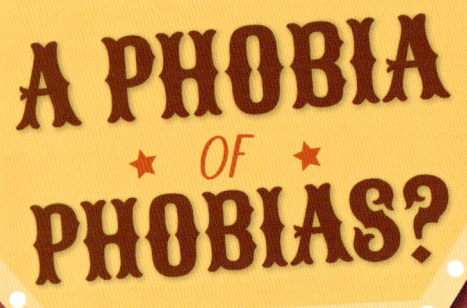

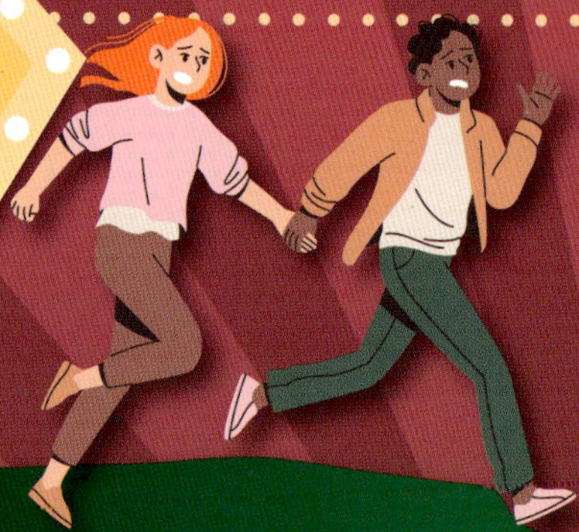

Have you been enjoying the show so far? Has anything scared you? Maybe you have become afraid of... becoming afraid?

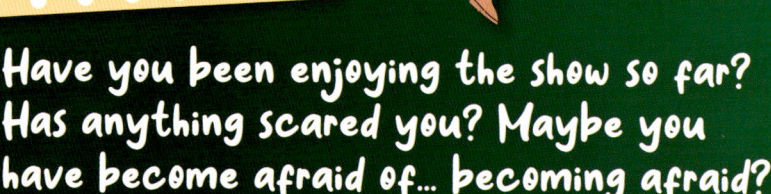

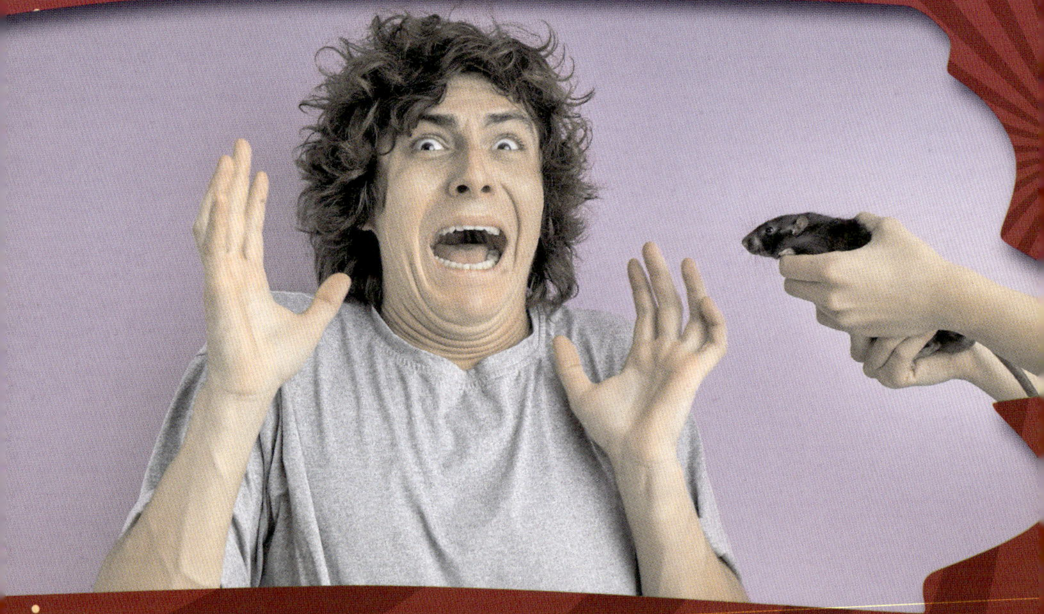

Can you feel that creeping into your stomach yet? You might not be afraid of anything that has been in our show, but maybe just the idea of being scared frightens you more than anything.

Some people with a phobia of phobias might be scared of feeling the physical signs of fear, such as a tightness in the chest.

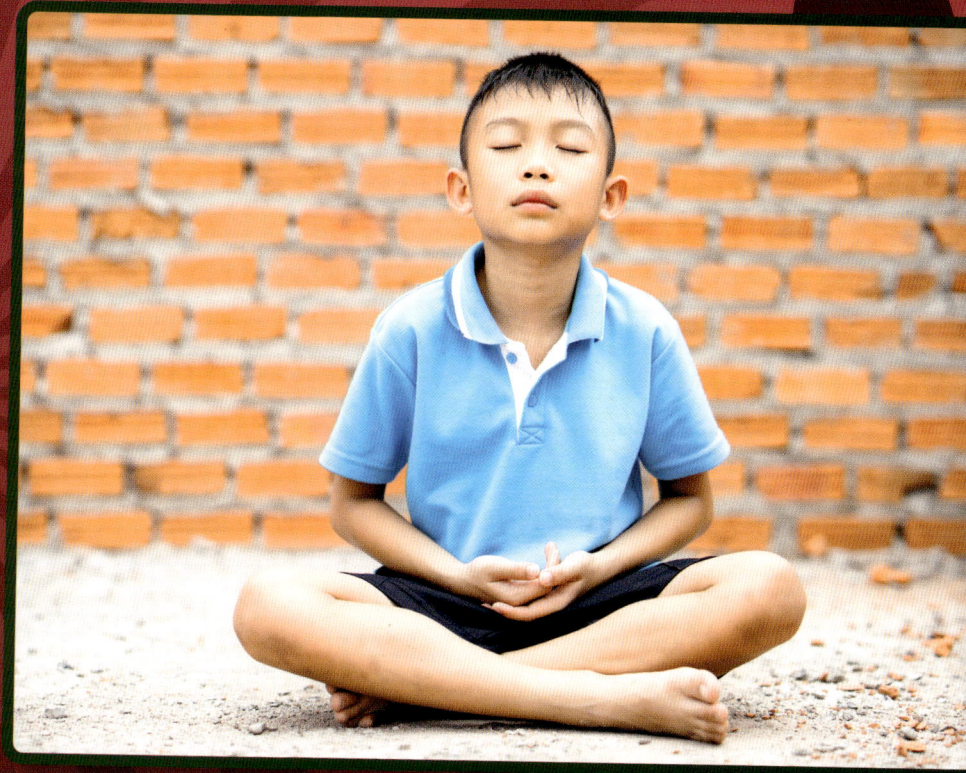

Unlike other phobias, worrying about being scared can actually bring on the phobia. However, people with this fear can try relaxing exercises such as slow breathing, yoga or talking about it with someone.

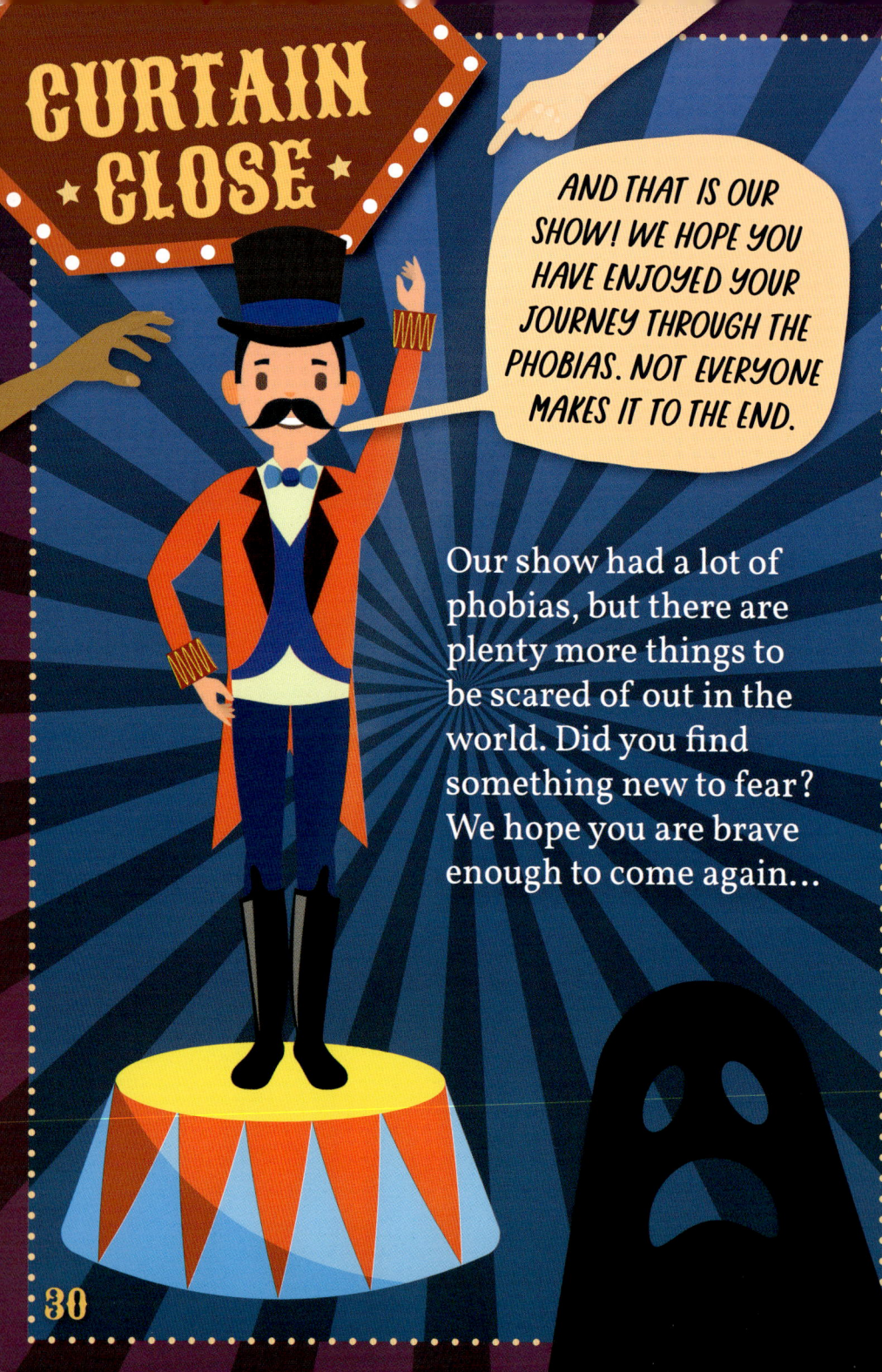

GLOSSARY

advise — to help someone make a choice

automatic — happening without being told to start

entertain — to do something that another person or group enjoys, usually as some sort of show

executed — killed as a punishment

hormone — chemicals in your body that tell cells what to do

ingredients — the parts of a recipe

orphanage — a place that takes care of children

vulnerable — being easy to attack or harm

INDEX

adrenaline 13–14

beards 8–9

clowns 26–27

itches 24–25

knees 10–11

Marilyn Monroe 22–23

nervous system 12, 15

teeth 16–17

witches 6–7

AN INTRODUCTION TO BOOKLIFE RAPID READERS...

Packed full of gripping topics and twisted tales, BookLife Rapid Readers are perfect for older children looking to propel their reading up to top speed. With three levels based on our planet's fastest animals, children will be able to find the perfect point from which to accelerate their reading journey. From the spooky to the silly, these roaring reads will turn every child at every reading level into a prolific page-turner!

CHEETAH
The fastest animals on land, cheetahs will be taking their first strides as they race to top speed.

MARLIN
The fastest animals under water, marlins will be blasting through their journey.
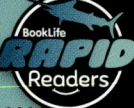

FALCON
The fastest animals in the air, falcons will be flying at top speed as they tear through the skies.
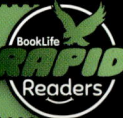